Rapid W

Motivation

Confidently Lose Weight Permanently with These Simple, Yet Powerful Mindset Shifts

By: Timothy Willink & Rapid Weight Loss Academy

Disclaimer

While all attempts have been made to verify the information provided in this publication, neither the author nor the publisher assumes any responsibility for errors, omissions, or contrary interpretations of the subject matter herein.

This book is for entertainment purposes only. The views expressed are those of the author alone and should not be taken as expert instructions of commands. The reader is responsible for his or her own actions.

Table of Contents

Introduction

In a world where we are surrounded by goofy gimmicks, "get-thin-quick" tricks, special work-out equipment, high-priced supplements, and tricked-out diet plans designed to all deliver quick results with little to no effort from us, we know this is rarely effective.

We don't need to take out a loan or mortgage our homes to be able to achieve our weight loss goals. The thing we need can't be bought or sold, but once you master it, it will be priceless.

We are talking about motivation!

A person could buy all the special work-out equipment the world has to offer, but it won't do a thing for them if they don't have the motivation to hop on it and use it.

A person can work with the best weight loss and nutrition specialists on the planet and have every supplement, diet plan, and special food at their disposal, but the numbers on their scale won't budge if they don't have the motivation to follow the plan as prescribed.

Weight loss, especially rapid weight loss, cannot be achieved without motivation.

This is the most important piece of the weight loss puzzle.

It might be easy to think, “But of course I’m motivated! I want to lose this weight, and I want to do it fast! I’m motivated because I want it.”

But wait a moment here. This is just a desire for the end result. This isn’t the motivation that will not only be helpful but will be *essential* for the rapid weight loss goals that you have. Desire just means you want something. Desire just means that something looks good to you.

What is motivation then? Motivation can be intrinsic or extrinsic, meaning it is either coming from within ourselves or from outside of ourselves, and they both have their place in leading us to success.

Desire plays its part in the motivational process, yes, but it doesn’t provide the energy and discipline needed to complete the motivational process. Don’t worry: that is what you will learn how to do in this book.

You know you have the desire, and if you’re like most people, you’ve probably had that desire for a long time.

About half of the population in the United States says they want to lose weight, but the percentage of these people that will actually meet their weight loss goal will fall far short. Why?

There are many reasons why people fall short of their weight loss goals, but most fall under the following categories:

- Goal-Setting Problems
- Workout Issues
- Personal Attitude Issues
- Diet Fantasy vs Reality
- Support System
- Lifestyle Fit
- Mental Health
- Adaptability

In order to be successfully motivated to meet your rapid weight loss goals- to be *truly motivated* to meet your rapid weight loss goals- you must first make a conscious choice to look at these categories and to commit to developing both the intrinsic and extrinsic motivations for each of them.

This requires being willing to look at each of these categories and to ask yourself the questions that may not be so easy to answer, but are necessary because your answers will be the way you will be able to successfully kick start your motivation to meet your rapid weight loss goals.

In the quest for weight loss, especially *rapid* weight loss, it is all too common for us to view the experience as being one of exclusive external change. After all, we are trying to change our external bodies, right? We want to see the weight of our external bodies shift and melt away. We want to be able to just make a few external adjustments in how we eat and how we move our bodies and then we want to see this magnificent external transformation that everyone that knows us will take a step back and gasp in astonishment at our accomplishments.

However!

While yes, external change is certainly a part of the process and an important one at that, there is more to it. It is true; you will not shed those unwanted pounds if you do not make some external changes in how and what you eat, and how you move your body. Where we go wrong, however, is in overemphasizing the external changes involved in weight loss and we almost always ignore the internal.

In order to see that magnificent transformation of rapid weight loss, we have to work on both the outside *and the inside*. We can't skip over a big part of the reason we got to this point, which is typically due to internal reasons. No one starts overeating, gorging on sweets, or laying around on the couch all day because they are at their peak mental and emotional condition.

As we pointed out before, there are a ton of gimmicks, tricks, supplements, and other “get-thin-quick” schemes out there, all dedicated to trying to make us feel like the only thing we need to hit our weight loss goals is this one single item we need to buy.

We all know that’s not correct; most of us know this because we’ve been through them all, and nothing seems to work the way it is advertised to.

There’s a reason for this, and that reason is why you are here, reading this book. Motivation.

Surrounding ourselves with all the weight loss gimmicks in the world won’t budge our waistlines, but the beauty of it is that once we figure out how to develop our internal motivations, we won’t need gimmicks anymore!

Building and maintaining your internal motivation is life changing, and this is a skill that transfers to all other areas of your life as well.

You’ve picked up the right book, and you’re on the right track. This is the beginning of the most effective rapid weight loss journey you’ve ever been on because you’re about to learn the simple, but incredibly effective methods for building a rapid weight loss plan that works for you, not against you.

Rapid Weight Loss Motivation *is* possible. You only need to keep reading to find out for yourself.

How to Get the Most out of This Book

It is my hope and desire that every single person that purchases this book will find their inner motivation to hit their rapid weight loss goals, but I know that there will be some that may not. I believe that if you use this book as it is intended, you will find success.

I suspect that if someone is to decide to just scroll through this book quickly, mining for little blurbs and bits that they think look easy or that they know they can quickly do, then that is what they will get. The easy way out. The path of least resistance.

However!

If someone is picking up this book with the intense desire to achieve their rapid weight loss goals, I suspect that that person will read this book in its entirety, start to finish, and will absorb the information and guidance that has been so painstakingly gathered here for them.

That person will reap the rewards. That person will reach their rapid weight loss goals.

This book is not offering an easy way out. This book is not offering a "quick fix" in the sense that you just need to swallow this pill or buy this one piece of equipment and you will be able to meet your rapid weight loss goals- no.

This book is offering you something much more tangible, much more realistic, much more life-changing, and much more powerful.

This book is offering you the way to dig in and unleash the power of your inner motivation so all your actions and efforts will be concentrated and your potential to meet your rapid weight loss goals will snowball as your inner motivation will push you successfully across the finish line.

You can use this book as an "easy" read that you simply scroll through while the TV blares in the background or you can use this book as the guidebook for your future. You can use this book to show you how to unleash the inner motivation that will drive you on your quest to not only meet your rapid weight loss goals, but also any other goal you are after in your life. Inner motivation is the vehicle that carries you on the road to success.

It is up to you to decide how successful you will be with this.

Are you ready to dig in and unleash the power of your inner motivation to meet your rapid weight loss goals?

Good. Let's do this!

Chapter 1: Plan Your Motivation

For just a moment, stop and imagine something with me. Let's imagine you were just told about a brilliant new opportunity to make your wildest dreams come true, and all you need to do to take advantage of it is to get to a specific location by a specific time.

You have the address for the location, but you do not know the exact route to get there. You have a general idea, but the clock is ticking; you want to be there to take advantage of this opportunity presented to you, and the pressure is on.

What will you likely do? Will you decide to A) plug in the address into your GPS and follow the instructions carefully in a safe but swift manner or B) decide to wing it and head off in the general direction (what you think is the general direction, anyway) in a fast and haphazard way?

Most people would choose A, right?

This holds true for any high-stakes goal. We all want to believe that we know how to get the results we're looking for, and we do all know the “general direction” but that is not good enough.

Most of us know and have always known what the standard advice is for people looking to lose weight. Eat less and move more. Watch your calories and get more exercise. Eat healthily and get active.

This is not inaccurate, of course. But it is only one piece of the puzzle. Not only is it just one piece of the puzzle, but its one piece of a rather large puzzle, and many of us have never seen the whole thing put together before.

We are going to put it together. We are going to look at the different areas that we have to plan out in order to hit our rapid weight loss goals. Just as we wouldn’t chance getting lost on the way to a major opportunity with a time limit, we aren’t going to leave our rapid weight loss journey up to chance, either.

There is a reason why so many of us have tried and failed to hit our rapid weight loss goals, and this is something we can fix. It is within our power to change; all we need is a plan that works **for us** rather than **against us**.

Chapter 2: Goal-Setting

The first category we need to look at what we have to make a plan for Goal-Setting. This may seem like a rudimentary step to take, as we know what goal you have in mind if you've picked up this book, right? Rapid weight loss.

Yes, we know the goal, but the goal is only where we hope to end up. The goal is not the road map to get there. This is where so many of us get off course on major goals like weight loss, especially weight loss with a ticking timer. We can have all the motivation in the world to reach a goal, but if we don't have the motivation to work the process to reach the goal, we will continue to spin our wheels fruitlessly.

This part of the planning process is a crucial first step to your rapid weight loss journey. Grab a notebook and a pen or take your notes digitally (although classic pen and paper have more of an impact psychologically than taking digital notes!)

Begin by considering what your exact weight loss goals are. Are you looking to be able to fit in a certain size clothing again? Do you want to see a specific number on your scale? Are you looking to reach the set weight range that your doctor gave you to get to buy your next appointment? What is going to be the thing that you are working towards specifically? This is very important. You can't be internally motivated to hit a goal if you don't have the specific goal outlined.

Be mindful of how you are writing your goal, as it will be helpful to refer back to this often. What is easier to keep up with? Something that depresses you or makes you anxious, like, "I want to lose 25 pounds of fat by August 1 because I feel like a beached whale," or something that makes you feel positive and hopeful, like, "My goal is to reach 135 pounds by August 1 so I will be healthier and more fit."

At first glance, this may not seem like such a big deal, but it is as simple as your goal either making you feel bad or feel good. We are working to develop our inner motivation, right? Will you be motivated to look at your goal and stay on your steady path if every time you open up your notebook you are depressed and anxious? No, you won't. You will experience a cascade of negative emotions, and this is not the best way to stay motivated to hit a big goal like rapid weight loss. All it will take is one bad day where you've hit a slump and aren't feeling your best, and then reading something negative that puts you even further down will seal your fate for that day.

So be sure to frame your goal in a positive light. Set a goal to work towards like a size you will become, vs how many sizes you have to "go down," and set a goal to work towards like the weight you want to be, vs how many pounds you have "to lose." This may not seem like a big deal, but every little bit of positive association you can build on your rapid weight loss journey will play a role in keeping that inner motivation going.

Below your main goal, be sure to list as many positive "side effects" as you can think of.

Perhaps it may be, "Once I reach my goal, I'll be able to run with my kids after school easier," or "Once I reach my goal, I'll feel more comfortable heading to the beach in the bikini I haven't worn in a long time," or "Once I reach my goal, my knee pain will get better." It's important to list all of the happy and positive ways that your life will change once you achieve your rapid weight loss goal, because every time you look at this list, your inner motivation will rev up.

These are your "reasons why," these will be the things you will call on to remember as you are sweating through a serious workout. These will be the reasons you will recall as you make a healthy dinner choice that you maybe would not have chosen before.

Remember, you want to build as many positive associations around your rapid weight loss goals as you can! Remember your reasons why.

Chapter 3: Workout Plans

Workout plans often come with workout issues. What do we mean by workout plan issues here? Do we mean that you simply haven't found the perfect trainer, or that you haven't purchased the right workout equipment for your at-home gym? No! Absolutely not.

All too often, people pursue weight loss strategies as if they are one size fits all. This could not be further from the truth!

Everyone has their strengths, their weaknesses, their likes, and their dislikes. There is no reason we shouldn't plan our workout strategies to reflect this!

To be able to tap into your inner motivation to achieve your rapid weight loss goals, you have to find the workout that works for *you* specifically.

Let's say your friend Jason was able to lose 25 pounds in a month just by picking up running in the mornings before work. He told you about it and you think, "wow! Yes, I'd like to lose 25 pounds in a month, too. I'm going to start running in the mornings before work!"

Well, this may go a few ways. Maybe you start running in the mornings before work and you

LOVE it! Maybe it is an incredible new morning routine for you and it makes you feel energetic and prepared for your day. You might end up thanking Jason for introducing you to this idea.

Or, maybe it is a difficult thing for you to do. Maybe you never have really been into running, and it always kind of bothers your knees and you end up cursing your run by the time the afternoon rolls around and your knees are screaming at you with every step. You might end up cursing Jason for introducing you to this idea!

With the first scenario, you're probably going to have no problem hopping out of bed each morning to put on those running shoes, right? But with the second scenario, you would probably be more likely to end up pushing that snooze button a few times too many!

The point here is that if you attempt to set up a workout plan that you hate just because someone else has seen excellent results from it, you will be setting yourself up for angst, unhappiness, and very likely- failure.

Remember what we did with the goal-setting? You need to do the same thing with your workout plans. You have to craft your workouts in such a way that they are associated with positivity and enjoyment, otherwise, it will always be too easy to find a reason or an excuse to skip out.

You can begin by making a list of all of the things that you love to do most. This list needs to be at least 10 items long. Now, go through the list, one by one, and inspect each thing to look at the physicality of it.

The beauty of this is that there are very often things that don't seem physical at all, that can often be tweaked to fit into a fitness plan!

For example, if you have "watch Netflix," on your list of the things you love to do most, and then you need to consider how to take that favorite thing of yours and how to turn it into a workout. A potential idea here might be to turn your Netflix time into a specific workout.

For example, perhaps when you want to binge watch your favorite show, maybe you only do it while walking on the treadmill or using the elliptical. Or maybe in order to watch the next episode, you build in a mini-sweat session into each episode break where you take 10 minutes to sweat it out with some serious aerobic activity, and then during the episode itself, you could be on your living room floor on a yoga mat doing Pilates.

Or maybe you have "hanging out with friends," as one of your favorite things to do. Great! Now, be sure to build your hangout time with friends into something that will be an enjoyable but effective workout. For example, maybe you gather your friends together for a 5-mile hike or an all-day climbing session at the state park.

The whole point here is that your workouts do not have to be and should not be torturous. If they are miserable and you hate the activity, how easy do you suppose it will be to maintain the internal motivation necessary to keep up with them?

If you answered "not very," you are right!

Once you have your list of at least ten of your favorite things to do in workout form you have set yourself up for success! The more fun and enjoyable you can set up your workouts to be, the more likely it is that you will remain consistent and motivated to do them, and that is a very important piece of the rapid weight loss puzzle!

Working out, moving your body, and building strength and agility should be fun! If your workouts are associated with pain and frustration, then it is not likely that you will keep up with them.

Build positive associations with moving your body and working out, and you won't find yourself making excuses to skip over this important part of your weight loss plan anymore.

Chapter 4: Personal Attitude

Personal attitude! First off, it is important to clarify what this means.

We are not talking about who you are as a person here and if you are a motivated go-getter or more of a slacker couch potato, or if you are outgoing or introverted. This is instead about what your personal attitudes are towards your weight loss goals.

We have alluded to how important it is to have a positive association with the various parts of your weight loss plan, but in this section, we will explain why.

The psychology on what a difference a positive attitude makes is settled. Studies show that the more positive of an attitude a person has, they are much more likely to reach their weight loss goals! In addition to this, positive attitudes are also associated with decreased anxiety and an improved mood, and anxiety and poor mood are both potential roadblocks to remaining consistent on your rapid weight loss journey.

So how can you be sure to cultivate a positive attitude around your rapid weight loss journey?

Time to pull out your notebook again! Just as you began to do in the goal setting section with listing the side-effects of reaching your goal, now you will take it a step further.

Have you ever heard of a vision board? It is a collage that a person makes of all of the things they want to achieve so they can actively visualize themselves achieving these things. Vision boards help because they are an easy touchstone for us to be reminded of what we are working towards. This will be very important in building and maintaining that inner motivation for your rapid weight loss.

For example, if one of your side effects of meeting your goal is to be able to run with your kids again, then you could put a picture on your vision board of you running with your kids before, or you could print out or even draw (depending on what kind of an artist you are!) a picture of a person running with their kids. If one of your side effects of meeting your goal is to wear a bikini to the beach, then put a picture of yourself up on the board in a bikini when you were at your goal size, or find a picture of someone that size in a bikini, being happy and confident at the beach.

This works on a few levels. Visual input is very important in reaching goals, and by building a vision board full of the positive side effects of your rapid weight loss, you are creating an effective way to stay on the right track.

Be sure to build your board with lots of positive associations and smiling faces. This board should make you smile and be happy with your rapid weight loss goals every single time you glance at it.

Incorporate your favorite colors, patterns, and textures. Make your vision board be something that when you look at it, you smile. Reinforcing the positive associations of your weight loss goals will reinforce your internal motivations.

Some people even decide to add in other senses to their vision board mix! There might be a scented candle you like to light near your vision board, or maybe a song or soundtrack you like to have to play while you look at it.

Incorporating additional senses can even give your vision board an additional boost since you can now listen to the songs or soundtrack in other places as well and it will remind you of your vision board, or you can light the same scented candle while taking a bath and it will remind you of your vision board. You can use that extra time to remember and reinforce your "reasons why."

You will want to hang your vision board somewhere that it will be easy to see often. You can hang it in your living room, in your bedroom, anywhere that it will be easy for you to check in with anytime you need to remind yourself why you are doing what you are doing on your rapid weight loss journey.

These are your motivations and your "reasons why."

Chapter 5: Diet Fantasy vs Reality

We have all been here before, right? We read about the latest fad diet or some new meal planning trend, and we run out to the grocery store, spend a few hundred dollars on all of these foods we don't usually eat, probably don't have any experience preparing, and maybe don't even like!

Fast forward a week later. How successful were we with this new diet?

When the diet we choose to follow is more fantasy than reality, we are setting ourselves up for failure. You're not going to suddenly love to eat the foods you hate, or suddenly have double the time it requires to prepare the special meal plans on the diet, so the diet fantasy fails.

Don't worry, this is a common experience. You're not alone!

However, yes. In order to reach your rapid weight loss goals, your diet will likely need to be modified.

The good news is this does not need to be an excruciating process! In fact, this process should be fun and exciting as you discover new foods, new ways to prepare your foods and learn how to incorporate foods that will help to reduce your appetite and improve your metabolic health so you can really kick start your rapid weight loss goals.

The planning phase for this will first require some serious honesty on your part. Begin by writing out all of the most favorite foods that you eat on a regular basis. What is typically found in your fridge and your pantry? If it's in your kitchen more often than not, it needs to be written down!

Next step, write out all of the times you've eaten at a restaurant or had taken out in the last month. Consult your bank statements if you need help remembering. This includes coffee shop runs and food trucks!

Now for the painful part. For every one of your most favorite foods that you eat on a regular basis at home, look up calorie counts either by looking at the packaging or googling it. Write out the calorie counts and the other pertinent nutritional info, such as how much fat, fiber, and protein are in each item.

Now it's time to do the same with your typical restaurant and takeout orders. Most places will offer their nutritional offer on a website somewhere, but if there is nothing available, just google the generic information on the internet, such as "chicken street tacos nutritional information," and use that.

This part of the planning process is very important because you can't be motivated to shift your diet choices if you don't have the awareness of what this shift will do for you in your weight loss journey.

If your favorite food list is full of low calorie, low fat, high protein foods, then you're done with this step! Congratulations. If you're like most other people, there will likely be some things that need to be looked at closer, and that is our next step.

For every favorite food item that you eat on a regular basis at home, you get to find the healthier, weight loss version of it. For many things, this is not necessarily a difficult thing to do. Healthier versions of even the most nutritionally depleted junk foods exist at most health food stores, or if you are good around the kitchen, you can google homemade healthy recipes at making your healthier versions at home. Not only do you need to replace your most favorite foods with healthier versions (so swap out those strawberry pop tarts and pick up some low calorie, low fat, strawberry fiber pastries from your grocery store!) but you also need to be sure that the old favorites leave your house. If things are unopened, you can consider donating them to local food pantries or aid organizations, or just drop off with a lucky friend!

Now, go through your favorite restaurants and takeout places. If you already order the healthiest, low fat, low-calorie item on their menu, then great! If you are not, you need to do your homework on what will be the best thing for you to order from each place and commit to ordering that thing.

It should not be a thing you hate, because choosing foods you hate will only backfire on you later. You won't be happy with your order, and you will be much more likely to decide to "cheat" later because you are unsatisfied, and that is not how you will meet your rapid weight loss goals!

Sugar is one of the biggest culprits in weight loss diet failures, and it is everywhere and in everything. If you have a love of sugar- as most of us do- then you need to plan for how you will avoid this.

Again, your diet shouldn't be something you despise and groan about following, so you need to do some clever planning to avoid any sugar binges that you might find yourself wanting to indulge in.

The fruit is a natural sugar source that has the additional advantage of containing many vitamins, minerals, and fiber that help to keep you in your peak condition to achieve your rapid weight loss goals. Lots of people have success with ensuring they have fresh fruit available to them at all times- in their car, in their bag, in their office, in their bedroom even! That way, when that sugar bug comes crying out to you for a calorie-laden candy bar, you can grab an orange or an apple instead.

This may not seem significant, but fruit sugar in its natural state is processed more easily by the body than the processed sugar that is found in sweet, sugary snacks. This holds true for many different foods. If you can, always opt for the natural, whole food over the processed, pre-packaged version. Swapping these out can have big effects on your waistline.

Now that you have swapped out your favorite foods at home and out for the healthiest versions, you have planned your diet for success and built your diet in a way that will be easy for you to remain internally motivated to stick with.

There are a variety of diets out there designed for weight loss, and they may work for different people in different ways. But for us, we all know that the best diet is the one that you actually do!

Chapter 6: Support System

Support systems. This is one of the most underrated aspects of meeting any goal, but especially for weight loss goals.

Why is it that people need support systems when pursuing weight loss goals? Well, there are a few reasons for this.

One obvious reason is for accountability's sake. If you decide to work with a nutritionist or a personal trainer, they are now a part of your support system. They will be there if you hit a roadblock or setback in your journey and will be able to help put you back on the path towards rapid weight loss. This will differ from your best friend who may not only be overly sympathetic with your setback, but they may even choose to reinforce your setback with a well-meaning offer to participate with you! For example, let's say you forget about the new order you've picked out for yourself at your favorite restaurant, and you ordered your high calorie, high fat, usual.

Understandably, when you realize this, you feel upset and disappointed with yourself, so you call up your friend to tell them about this and then what do they do? Maybe say, "Oh man, I fell off my diet wagon last night too! Eh, since we've already broken our diets, let's meet up at our favorite frozen yogurt place and have a cheat day together!"

This obviously would not be as helpful as would the likely response from a professional support person, such as your nutritionist. That conversation would look a little different!

Rather than decide to double down on the disruption, your nutritionist would be more likely to respond to a slip-up with something like this:

"Oh! Well, sometimes that will happen, but that's alright, you can get back on track. In order to compensate for the additional calorie intake from last night, let's talk about a few adjustments you can make today to keep moving towards your rapid weight loss goals!"

Obviously, we can see which one will be more helpful in supporting our internal motivations.

This is not to say that there isn't an important place for social support in your rapid weight loss journey, because there absolutely is!

One of the most effective ways to maintain your motivation during your weight loss journey is to include others that are on a similar journey in your social circle. By being around others that are also on a weight loss journey, you are creating informal accountability between you and them, which is important because it can be celebrated when you are being successful and it can be an important nudge to get back on track when you find yourself slipping behind.

Some people even like to make fun and informal contests with their friends about who can reach their personal goals first, which can add a spirit of competition to it which can be incredibly motivating for some! If you are one of these people that are very motivated by competition but you don't have any friends that are interested, you can consider reaching out on social media such as Twitter and Facebook to see if there's anyone that will participate with you.

There are also people who even choose to take this fun competition a step further and make a side wager on who will meet their weight loss goals first! Anything that motivates and keeps things fresh and fun works!

This sort of social support is not just fun, but it's also incredibly motivating, particularly if you make the challenge public! Having people rooting for you and monitoring your progress can really make the difference in a moment where you are considering slacking off on an important workout or indulging in something that you know isn't going to help you meet your weight loss goals.

Here's another interesting bonus to the group support/fitness challenge dynamic. Studies have found that the person who initiates and coordinates the social support/fitness challenge group tends to be even *more* successful in reaching their weight loss goals! This would be extra helpful for someone who is on a rapid weight loss journey.

If you are an extreme introvert and cannot possibly imagine reaching out for a social support system, you can fake one to still reap some of the psychological benefits!

Build your own personal blog or use a notebook to journal in, but document your weight loss plans and your journey. Be sure to comment daily on your progress. Be sure to encourage yourself to keep going when you've hit a rough spot, and celebrate your successes and victories! Keep yourself accountable.

Whatever path you choose to go, plan carefully and don't forget to set up your support systems. Support systems will be important both in building and in maintaining your rapid weight loss motivation!

Chapter 7: Lifestyle Fit

Lifestyle fit.

One of the major reasons why people fail to maintain their rapid weight loss motivation is because they have chosen weight loss plans that do not fit into their lifestyle.

When this happens, it's like trying to swim upstream- and it will get old very fast.

One example of this might be with workout choices. If you decide that running on the beach in the soft sand is going to be your daily morning workout, but you live an hour away from the beach and the only way to make it there for your workout then back home and to work on time is to wake up at 3am, then that will probably not work. This probably won't be sustainable.

You might really want to make it work, and you might really *try* to make it work, but eventually, the sleep deprivation and the stress of this choice will likely damage your efforts. However romantic it may sound, it just does not fit into your lifestyle.

Rather than attempt to overhaul your lifestyle in a way that is less likely for you to be consistent with, consider the ways you can fit your weight loss goals into your current lifestyle. Be realistic in what you can do, but be creative!

Do you work a desk job? You could consider setting a timer for every half hour where you get yourself up and out from behind your desk to take a brisk walk out to the hallway, where you could maybe do thirty squats or fifty jumping-jacks or whatever the particular thing you could find yourself doing may be. Or maybe you could go run up and down the back flight of stairs a few times. You don't have to quit your desk job; you just have to find creative ways to continue your rapid weight loss goals at work!

Or perhaps you work in a job where a part of each week is a special treat in the breakroom- maybe donuts or some other high calorie, high fat, sugary pastry. If you know when this is coming and you know you will want some, it may not work out that you can simply avoid the breakroom or your coworkers coming by to chat about them, so you could instead make a modification in another part of your day's diet or fitness routine to accommodate this one treat.

Another idea would be to bring your own "special treat" from home that is a healthier version of one of your favorite foods that you already replaced out. This way you are still participating in an advantageous social experience at work, you are still getting a bit of a "special treat," and you aren't finding yourself feeling guilty or like you've set your rapid weight loss goals back.

You don't- and should not- attempt to overhaul every facet of your life all at once, even while working towards a significant goal like rapid weight loss. Attempting to do too much all at once can backfire, and people sometimes find that when this happens, their weight loss goals are given up on as they find themselves overwhelmed with all of the lifestyle changes.

There are ways to make small, but meaningful tweaks to your lifestyle that will deliver big results towards your weight loss goals. Remember, you want this to be a positive experience that you will not lose motivation for!

Look at your daily transportation. This is one of the easiest tweaks to make in daily lifestyle choices.

Do you park in one of the closest spots to the building you work at? Start parking in the spot that is furthest away so you get a few extra steps in. Do the same everywhere you go in your car. Instead of parking on the same street, park around the corner. Instead of parking in the parking garage, park across the street.

These are small tweaks that still fit within your lifestyle.

Just as with diets, lifestyle tweaks only work if you can make them work for you! If you try to change things so drastically that you know you will never be able to keep up with them, then you are sabotaging yourself and your rapid weight loss motivation.

Chapter 8: Mental Health

Mental health is no different than physical health. If you have a physical health injury such as a sprained ankle, you would need to modify your weight loss plans to account for that, right?

No one would expect you to go run up and down a flight of stairs several times a day with a sprained ankle, regardless of how many calories you might burn doing so.

Mental health is the very same. There are some mental health circumstances that are associated with being overweight, such as depression and low self-esteem. If you are experiencing this sort of negative mental health headspace, then maintaining your motivations for rapid weight loss will be like trying to clean your house in the middle of a tornado.

There are many avenues you can down to access mental healthcare that will support you in your weight loss goals and many people start by seeing their primary care doctor for a mental health referral.

If you are not interested in seeing a professional, there are new peer-supported mental health services available for free where you can call a number or enter a chat room and talk directly to people called “listeners” who are thoughtful listeners and able to help provide a soundboard for your issues and concerns. Examples of these include websites such as “7 Cups” and “Blah Therapy,” which you can find by typing directly into Google.

There are also a variety of ways you can take your mental health care in your own hands, including the use of creative methods such as creating art or journaling. Creative pursuits have positive mental health effects such as decreased stress, improved self-esteem, and emotional release.

Boosting the way you feel about yourself and the way you are feeling, in general, will always have a positive effect on your internal motivations, and because both stress and self-esteem have a direct impact on weight loss, this positive effect is magnified.

Watch how you talk about yourself, because guess what? **You are listening**!

If you tell yourself daily that you are lazy and unable to hit your rapid weight loss goals, then that is what you will carry with you. That will be your truth.

Instead of that, keep your headspace positive and encouraged. Every time you look in the mirror, use some positive self-talk: “You’re doing great! Look at you, on the way to <insert

positive weight loss goal side effect here>. You are working so hard, this is great!"

It may seem a little silly at first, but please understand that your mental health and your headspace is an incredibly important part of how successful you will be in building and maintaining the internal motivation to move towards your rapid weight loss goals.

Whatever story you tell yourself that will be your story. Are you telling yourself that you are lazy and will fail? Then that will be your story. Are you telling yourself that you are working hard to meet your rapid weight loss goals? Then that will be your story.

Always work to reframe your story in the way you want to see it play out. Be an active player, not a passive participant!

In order to build and maintain the internal motivation that you will need to meet your rapid weight loss goals, getting your mental health in peak condition will be essential. This is a piece of the puzzle that will also go on to positively affect all other areas of your life, as well!

Chapter 9: Adaptability

Adaptability, the enemy of inflexibility. How do you know if you are adaptable or inflexible?

Well, let's see. Consider the following scenario: If a friend calls to tell you that they changed the restaurant reservation at the last moment and you are now meeting at a new location, do you A) say, "Oh, okay, that's fine. See you soon!" and then continue getting ready to go out, or do you B) say, "Oh. Okay, I guess so. See you soon." And then continue getting ready but now you are in a state of angst because your plans changed at the last minute and you HATE that.

Choice B would be a good indicator of some personal inflexibility. The inverse to personal inflexibility is adaptability, and this will be an important aid in building and maintaining motivation for your rapid weight loss.

Adaptability is the ability to easily move into and out of situations and scenarios, even if they are completely unexpected and require an entire shift of effort or plans.

The ability to adapt to your situation is one that can save you a ton of emotional distress in the long run, and as it pertains to motivation for rapid weight loss, it is huge.

Any number of scenarios can crop up in your day that might throw off something like your workout plan for the day, or your diet choice for dinner, and you will have two options: You can be personally inflexible and allow it to cause a stressful situation internally in which you may find yourself giving up for the day, or you can be adaptable, and choose to shift your perspective and your plans and problem solve a way to work through the disruption.

For example, maybe you had planned to go for a swim at the local pool after work, and you had your suit and towel packed and ready to go. You arrive at the pool only to see it's been closed for the day. You can let this be the "reason" or the excuse you give up on your workout for the day, or you can instead embrace your adaptability and shift your perspective.

Okay, you can't swim. That's alright, what else is nearby? Maybe there's an indoor climbing gym, and you can swing by there and get some climb time in instead.

If you find yourself going down the path of inflexibility and saying something like, "well, looks like I can't work out today because of this!" then use this as a great time to practice some self-talk.

You can think of self-talk like this: how would you talk to a small child that just found out their favorite playground was under construction? Would you say, "Oh, looks like you don't get to play today? That sucks," or would you look for comparable alternatives so the small child can still get some playtime in?

Maybe it would sound something like this: "Oh, looks like you can't play at this playground today. That's okay, where else can you play? There's a playground a few blocks here, you can play there!"

We owe it to ourselves to treat ourselves kindly, just as we would a small child that's been disappointed because their favorite playground is under construction. The more you can do this, the better chances that you won't decide to "punish" yourself by forgoing the plan altogether to wallow in your disappointment.

A quick side note here about preparing for adaptability. In the scenario described above, you would have to shift quickly from a plan of swimming to a plan of climbing, but you only had your swimsuit and a towel with you, and you are wearing your work clothes. In order to be truly adaptable, you need to be prepared. An easy way to do this would be to always have an extra pair of stretchy, comfortable workout clothes and sneakers handy in a bag or in the trunk of your car. Be prepared to adapt!

Chapter 10: Live Your Motivation

So here you are! You've made it through the planning stages. You've done your homework. Now you are truly prepared to begin working towards your rapid weight loss goals.

One of the major factors that often sets people back on their weight loss goals is lack of motivation, and specifically, internal motivation.

There are many ways to build and maintain internal motivation. The first step was to plan out what your game plan would be on your rapid weight loss journey and to work on building and maintaining your internal motivation.

Now it is time to **live** your motivation!

One of the most powerful things to remember regarding internal motivation is that it is not finite. There is not just only so much of it that each person has before it fades away, and it isn't something that needs to be chased down in order to find success.

Motivation is a skill. Just as with any other skill, the more you practice it, the better you will become at it!

This is not an “I did it one time, and now I’m good,” sort of skill. It requires repetition, but just as with any skill you want to have, you just keep working on it and improving as you go. It is like building any muscle- you’ve got to work it out to make it stronger and more powerful.

To live your motivation on your rapid weight loss journey, it is often necessary for many to begin the first few days to a week (you know yourself best-how long will it take you to build up this muscle?) of your weight loss journey being as strict and disciplined with yourself as you can be.

The idea here is to create these positive habits so your mind and body will be able to follow your rapid weight loss plan with ease.

Resistance is going to happen. It is just a part of the human experience, so that is why we begin the path to rapid weight loss motivation with the planning of positive associations and positive head space so that this resistance will be easier to overcome.

The psychology behind this is important because, in pursuit of any endeavor, there will be resistance. Anything that is difficult to do and requires a significant amount of effort, our minds will come up with excuses to back out of. That is why the more we can build our weight loss plans to be a positive experience, the easier they will be to continue on with.

When our weight loss goals are tied into the experience of pain and pressure, they then are easier for us to back out of and push off for another day. Who wants to do something that is painful?

For most of us, this is not motivating.

Building a plan for our rapid weight loss goals that is full of positive associations is the way to ensure that internal motivation can be maintained.

The best and most comprehensive weight loss plan is absolutely useless if a person does not do it. The best of intentions will never get us to meet our goals.

However, if we can create a positive and fulfilling plan that makes us feel good while we are doing it, then that internal motivation will not be hard to find!

In setting up your rapid weight loss goals and associating them to the positive results that you are wanting to see in your life, such as being able to run after your children again, or being able to fit in a favorite outfit, allows the mind to be excited about the endeavor.

This positive headspace is what can make all of the difference when it comes to deciding if you're going to work your plan today or have a "cheat day."

Think of it like this: If your rapid weight loss plan isn't something that is associated with pain and misery, then why would you want to "cheat" on it? The answer? You won't!

The reason we have this idea in our society that diets are meant to be "cheated on" is because we usually think of a diet as something that is inherently negative. Let me assure you, it is not, and it never needs to be!

When we build weight loss plans that include workouts and foods that we hate, then we are building weight loss plans that will zap our motivations to do them. We are setting ourselves up for failure.

No one wants to do the things they hate. No one wants to eat the foods they hate. This holds true in every single aspect of our lives.

What's your favorite thing to do? Do you love to sing in the shower? Do you love to paint your nails? Do you love to go shopping?

Have you ever lost your motivation to do these things?

Have you ever felt like you just couldn't find the energy or motivation to do these things that you love?

Of course not! Because when we are doing things we love, we don't need to find our motivation. We do them because we enjoy them, and this is the surefire way to build a rapid weight loss plan that you won't need to "find" motivation for!

Living your motivation means that you have structured your weight loss plans in such a way that keeping them feels good! You should LOVE your rapid weight loss goals! You should LOVE the workouts you have designed. You should be EXCITED to tweak your lifestyle so you hit your rapid weight loss goals.

Anything less than this is going to be a source of stress and misery. This is the opposite of motivation, and we know that we need the motivation to keep pushing to reach our rapid weight loss goals.

Let the power of your own internal motivation **work for you**!

Conclusion

Motivation, especially internal motivation, is a very powerful thing. Most people are motivated by doing things that feel good. We are motivated by pleasure, and we are motivated by reward.

How is it then that we often set big goals for ourselves, such as rapid weight loss goals that are associated with nothing but pain and misery? Why do we make diet plans to eat foods that we hate? Why do we set up workout strategies that we know in advance we will hate to do? Why do we assume that doing things we hate will be the most effective way to reach our goals?

This is an interesting situation that most of us put ourselves in when it comes to weight loss goals. We think the only path there is one of pain and misery. So, when it is painful and miserable, what do we do?

We "cheat," we decide we don't want to do that today, or even worse, we quit! No one likes to be miserable, right?

That is why a truly successful weight loss plan or strategy cannot be full of things that are painful and misery-inducing. All of the supplements, workout equipment, fitness aids, etc., won't be able to make up for the fact that if something is associated with pain and misery, our brains will fight like heck to keep from having to do it!

We have to stop telling ourselves that the only way to achieve significant weight loss is to put ourselves in distress. The easiest way to do this is to build a weight loss plan that is full of positive associations. We want associations that are positive. We want associations that feel good! Then the question won't be, how do I make myself do this, but rather- *why wouldn't I do this???*

Now that you've read the steps to building a rapid weight loss plan that you love, you will be able to apply these principles to other areas of your life, as well.

When we associate positively to something, we decrease the angst and the struggle that surrounds it. We reduce the stress, and we increase the likelihood that we will continue with it.

Build positive associations in all that you do, and continue to find ways to reframe any negative headspace you may find yourself in. Build a vision board that speaks to you. Let your "reasons why" lead the way.

Be realistic in your weight loss goals, and remember that an adaptable mindset is one of the most powerful tools you will have at your disposal during your rapid weight loss journey. Sometimes the playground may be closed; be adaptable and always continue on with your personal goals even if your plans have to shift a bit.

Yes, you need to make an effective diet and exercise plan, but it should not be comprised of things you hate and will try to avoid like the plague.

Find and/or build your social support systems. Whether they're professional nutritionists and fitness trainers, or just a group you get together of Facebook friends that are working towards similar goals, this kind of support can be priceless when it comes to sticking with weight loss plans.

The most effective rapid weight loss plan is always going to be the one you do, so build yours the way it works best for you, and you'll never have to worry about "finding" the motivation to stick with it ever again!

FREE BONUS

P.S. Is it okay if we overdeliver?

I believe in overdelivering way beyond our reader's expectations. Is it okay if I overdeliver?

Here's the deal, I am going to give you an extremely valuable cheatsheet of "Accelerated Learning"...

What's the catch? I need to trust you... You see, my team and I wants to overdeliver and in order for us to do that, we've to trust our reader to keep this bonus a secret to themselves. Why? Because we don't want people to be getting our ultimate accelerated learning cheatsheet without even buying our books itself.

Unethical, right?

Ok. Are you ready?

Simply Visit this link:
http://bit.ly/acceleratedcheatsheet

Everything else will be self explanatory after you've visited: http://bit.ly/acceleratedcheatsheet

We hope you'll enjoy our free bonuses as much as we've enjoyed preparing it for you!

CPSIA information can be obtained
at www.ICGtesting.com
Printed in the USA
BVHW071016090919
557930BV00003B/568/P